I0414093

There Is Hope!

Surviving Merkel Cell Carcinoma

By: Peter D. Jepson, ChFC®

There is Hope! — Surviving Merkel Cell Carcinoma

© 2019 Copyright by Peter D. Jepson

ISBN: 978-1-63073-292-9

Faithful Life Publishers • North Fort Myers, FL 33903
888.720.0950 • info@FaithfulLifePublishers.com
FaithfulLifePublishers.com

All rights reserved. No part of this publication may be reproduced, stored in a retrieval system, or transmitted in any form or by any means—electronic, mechanical, photocopy, recording, or any other—except for brief quotations in printed review, without the prior permission of the publisher.

Published in the United States of America
23 22 21 20 19   1 2 3 4 5

For Dylan—

I am the man that your love made,
and you are my gift to the world.

TABLE OF CONTENTS

ACKNOWLEDGMENTS

Without God this book would not be possible. His blessings have provided me with so many precious moments in life. Through my journey with Merkel Cell Carcinoma He renewed what little hope I had and restored my belief in the power of prayer.

Many individuals who contributed to the stories in this book did so in anonymity. Others like my friend and Physician Assistant Beth McDonough, Riverchase Dermatology, Dr. David Ritter and staff, all the doctors, nurses and technicians who cared for me during my journey, and the Skin Cancer Foundation are recognized and receive my gratitude for their expertise in treatment and advocacy in skin cancer.

Much gratitude also goes to Mollie Page, my editor at Print Page, who helped me write the book, did most of the research, and worked with all the creatives, media, and publisher to get it printed and into the hands of readers.

I'd also like to thank Julie Koester, Patrick Blake Renda, and Ed Clay with Dragon Horse Media for their brilliant cover design and ongoing marketing assistance.

To Jim Wendorf of Faithful Life Publishers, our chance meeting was most fortuitous.

I also want to acknowledge the generosity of my friends and neighbors at Miromar Lakes, as well as George DeSantis, Michael Reynolds, Scott Chapman, Dave Georges, George Leamon, Mary Glenn, Bob Lovell, Janet Lovell, Ross Martin, Steve Erchowsky, Mitch Mann, Amber Jepson, and my dear brother Steve Jepson. All my friends and clients who have touched my life, you gave me the courage to share my story.

And to Cori the mother of my son, your support and compassion helped me see the bigger picture in life.

— Peter D. Jepson

Chapter 1:

Alone but Not Afraid

I t's funny how certain songs can influence our feelings
and change the way – if only momentarily – we see and
think about a situation.

I can't remember what songs are playing on the radio
most mornings but I remember hearing the song "Free
Fallin'" by Tom Petty and the Heartbreakers on the car
radio the morning I drove to my first radiation therapy
treatment.

Lucky for me the next song was "I Won't Back Down,"
another Petty classic. And in a split second, I was no longer
free falling. I became a warrior and was determined to
"stand my ground!"

2018 was a nightmare, to say the least. Diagnosed with
Merkel Cell Carcinoma in early April, followed by surgery
to remove a tumor on my temple that left my face looking
like a patchwork quilt of stitches, I was now facing two
months of radiation therapy treatments and an unknown
future.

It was July 10, 2018, another hot summer morning in
Southwest Florida. My son, Dylan and I had just spent the
Fourth of July together. A typical 16-year old boy, he was

more interested in lighting fireworks and eating lots of pizza than my next step in this damn cancer journey.

Cancer doesn't give you many choices. It's not like a box of jelly beans. You can at least share a box of jelly beans. Who wants to share their journey through cancer?

Radiation was what the doctor ordered, and that's where I was going on a muggy Tuesday morning. Alone, but with courage as my companion.

"There ain't no easy way out," I sang this line of the song as I locked the car door and proceeded to walk across the puddle-ridden parking lot to receive my first radiation therapy treatment.

Everyone Has an Origin Story

Damn the Torpedoes by Tom Petty and the Heartbreakers came out in 1979. I was in my final year of college, studying Economics at the University of Minnesota. Well, I was partying more than studying but that's to be expected. I remember buying the album and listening to it over and over. My favorite song on it was "Even the Losers," because, well you know, they get lucky sometimes.

I was born in the late summer of 1956 in Northfield, Minnesota. Our family moved around Minnesota and South Dakota until arriving in Detroit Lakes, Minnesota, when I was 14 years old.

In high school I spent most of my time on the water: boating, waterskiing, and hanging out with friends. Detroit Lakes is about 50 miles east of Fargo, North Dakota, and nowhere near Detroit.

There were lakes everywhere, though. Skiable lakes! By the 10th grade, I had mastered slalom skiing and was determined to be a barefoot master one day.

My father was a veterinarian. But running a business was tough for him and the family hit hard times in the 1950s causing him to leave the work he loved.

During most of my childhood my father worked as a meat packing inspector for the state. He was the most hated man in the meat packing and slaughterhouse industry because he refused to take bribes. We moved a lot in those days because it was the only way he could get a pay grade raise. But these relocations might have also been fueled by his reputation as a hard-nosed inspector.

My mother was a serious woman who rarely smiled. She was sad but not clinically speaking. My older brother, Tommy, had died from leukemia when he was four years old. She never recovered. In my last month of high school, the heartbreak finally overwhelmed her and she had a nervous breakdown from crying all those years.

Shortly after the death of President George H.W. Bush in 2018, a letter surfaced that he wrote to his mother about the great grief he felt after losing his daughter, Robin, to leukemia at age three. When I read it, I was reminded of the pain my mother must have endured for so many years.

Steve, my younger brother, and I were polar opposites as kids. We'd play outside everyday as kids, though, regardless of whether there was snow on the ground or a cloud of cicadas on the horizon. We'd race to the lakes during the summer and swim for as long as we could.

We were kids of the 1970s: no seatbelts or sunscreen necessary. And I was the prototypical Minnesota boy: blond hair with fair skin and lots of freckles.

Steve had astigmatism and even though he wore corrective glasses, the condition prevented him from playing sports or moving too rapidly. He was always six paces behind me wherever we went. Later in life, he was almost killed in a car accident. I don't know whether his sight issues had anything to do with it. It's not a question you ask.

Money was tight in our family when I was young. My father was not good at managing our finances and after years of struggling, my mother finally took control of all the money. She was very frugal and kept notes on everything from when to replace the dryer to how much to save each week until we could buy a new one.

My mother was a Lutheran but converted to the Church of Jesus Christ of Latter-day Saints when I was in high school. I think an incident when I was picked up by the police for being rowdy with friends and had to call her to come and get me might have motivated her conversion.

When she arrived at the police station, she walked right up to me and in front of everyone said, "Peter, you've sinned!" She made me attend church and pray beside her for six months. I was never on the wrong side of the law again.

As a young man, I was cripplingly shy around girls. And probably stupid, too. Well, one stupid and very pubescent thing I did was find the courage to ask the prettiest girl in school to prom and then never show up. I should go back and apologize to her, someday.

In 1975 I enrolled in classes at the University of Minnesota and began my studies to be a dentist like my grandfather. Within a year, I switched majors because I didn't like chemistry. I also found out that dentists have a high suicide rate.

When I returned to school my sophomore year, I enrolled in economics and thrived. For the next three years, I performed at the top of my class and in 1979 I graduated with a Business Administration Degree.

During my last year in college, I worked in construction – laying bricks mostly – and was making good money as a union member. I had a fast boat, great car, and with money in my pocket and a dark tan, was finding dating much easier too.

Like bikers or NASCAR fans, there's also a singular and unique culture of people that thrives on life on the water. I was born a Virgo, which is an Earth sign, but water runs in my veins. If it can be done on, with or behind a boat, I've done it!

I guess that's why I ended up in Florida.

The History of Merkel Cell Carcinoma

Cancer is a complex medical subject. It's not a virus and you can't get rid of it with chicken soup. It's more like rust or mold, except each type has a unique origin, diagnosis, treatment and prognosis.

The Merkel cell was first identified in 1875 by Freidrich Sigmund Merkel, a German Histopathologist. It may sound unconventional but his research included staining the skin of geese and ducks. He was later able to demonstrate a set of unique touch cells in the snouts of pigs. Through this primitive research he found that a unique set of cells reside at the dermoepidermal junction and near nerve fibers. Merkel postulated that the cells acted as mechanoreceptors in all animals.

But it wasn't until 1972, when a surgical pathologist named Cyril Toker found what he called "Toker's trabecular carcinoma of the skin." After many microscopic studies, Toker and his colleagues were able to identify dense-core neuroendocrine granules within the tumor cells, which they assumed were from Merkel cells.

Over time, research has found that Merkel Cell Carcinoma (MCC) occurs when there is a reduced immune function, which may be exacerbated by the presence of polyomavirus. However, the only undisputed and a major contributing factor of this cutaneous malignancy is exposure to ultraviolet radiation – i.e., the sun.

Other contributing factors are also being studied including the role of polyomavirus, which is found in 80% of MCC tumors. It's a rather benign virus, as viruses go. Possibly caught in childhood through respiratory secretions, the polyomavirus is naturally occurring and tends to stay latent in most hosts throughout life. However, when MCV (Merkel cell polyomavirus) is present in a host with an immunocompromised system, the risk of developing Merkel Cell Carcinoma is much greater.

In many Latin American countries, MCC has been linked to arsenic exposure in those who live in areas with naturally elevated levels of arsenic in the drinking water. Unfortunately, MCC data in Latin American countries is scarce because of a shortage in research funding and physician awareness of diagnosis and treatment options.

In 1988 there were 400 cases confirmed worldwide. Today, it is estimated that over 60,000 people have been diagnosed with MCC.

A Few Words on Melanoma

Like most people, I thought melanoma was the worst type of skin cancer until I was diagnosed with MCC.

Melanoma and MCC are both aggressive skin malignancies. However, according to the Skin Cancer Foundation about 2,500 cases of MCC are reported each year compared to more than 178,000 cases of melanoma.

Merkel cells are located in the top layer of skin and are very close to nerve endings. Melanoma affects melanocytes, the cells that protect skin and turn the pigment brown when exposed to sun.

Other differences include tumor location, sex and age of patient. In most melanoma cases, the malignancy is located on the trunk; while MCC tumors are more likely located on the head or neck. More men acquire MCC than women.

The average age of a melanoma patient is 57, while MCC tends to appear in patients (mostly men) over age 70.

MCC also has a higher likelihood of lymph node involvement.

Survival rates are much different, too. After one year, the survival rate is 92.9% for patients with melanoma and only 57.7% for those with MCC.

Chapter 2:

The Land of Sun and Fun

There may be 10,000 lakes in Minnesota, but there are 1,500 miles of navigable beaches and inland waterways in Florida. Plus, no winters! That was enough to convince me that Florida was where I wanted to start my post-college adult life.

Adulting was fun in Florida, too! I scored a job taking yearbook photos of students during the day and bartended during the evenings. One day, a bar patron told me I could make $6,000 a month selling water softener systems for Culligan.

For five years I sold water softener systems in Fort Myers, Florida. The town was booming during the 1980s, and new homeowners clambered for the best water treatment systems. The water in Florida is, how shall I say it, kind of gross and many new home wells are only about 50 feet deep.

During my Culligan days I'd typically travel door to door. Needless to say, I've been bitten by several dogs and chased off properties by more than one jealous or suspicious spouse. But I was also the top salesman every year during my employment with Culligan.

You tend to grow a thick skin when doing door-to-door sales. This quality helped me greatly when I decided to take a risk and become a financial planner.

It was the late '80s and the economy was on fire! The Feds let the interest rates fall a bit and oil prices fell, too. Investing and traveling were American's newest past times. As a financial planner, it was easy to help people build wealth so they could enjoy life more.

In my lifetime I've found that if you have money you have a greater sense of freedom and control of your life.

The Face of the Enemy

The call came in the afternoon. I had been a patient of Riverchase Dermatology for a few years and knew the staff well. Most visits to a dermatologist for a 60-something-year-old man who spent his free time water skiing and boating are pretty standard – lots of sun damage inevitably meant lots of basal cell lesion removals using liquid nitrogen. And mine were mostly on the face.

Like most water junkies growing up on the water, I opted for baby oil over sunscreen. The objective was to get and nurture a deep dark tan. And even though I was a fair-skinned boy from Minnesota, my skin eventually adapted over the years and stayed a nice toast color.

I had already experienced Mohs surgery to treat a squamous cell lesion on my neck so I was anticipating another Mohs-necessary diagnosis when I answered the call.

"Pete?" I recognized the voice as Beth McDonough, the Physician Assistant at Riverchase Dermatology who has a great sense of humor. She had taken a biopsy of what I thought was a small cyst on my temple the week prior.

"Hey Beth, what's up?" I asked as I slid off my chair at the country club and quickly moved across the room to a quieter corner.

"Pete. It's not squamous," she said and then quickly added, "and it's not basal either."

"Oh. What's left, melanoma?" I asked.

"No, Pete. Worse than melanoma," said Beth, whose voice was soft and trembling now.

"What do you mean?" I asked as I sat down in a chair nearby and looked up at the face of my buddy across the room. He gave me the thumbs up hand motion, but I shook my head and dropped my eyes to the floor.

"Merkel Cell, Pete," she answered.

"What's that?" I asked.

"The worst kind," she answered.

Over the years, I had encountered many clients and friends who were diagnosed with melanoma. One client even had part of his jaw removed. Was I about to lose part of my face? I thought melanoma was the end of the skin cancer spectrum. Now I had just found out there was an even more dire level – the worst-kind level!

"What do I do?" I asked Beth. My heart was racing and I suddenly felt dizzy.

"We're going to schedule you for surgery, Pete. It's got to be removed fast," said Beth. "I'll take care of everything. You'll get a call from the surgeon's office tomorrow with details. Don't worry, Pete. We're going to get this tumor out of you."

Tumor! She's calling it a tumor. I could barely breath.

"Pete! Did you hear me?" Beth's voice was louder now. "It's going to be ok."

"Ok, Beth. The surgeon. Tomorrow. Ok, Beth. Good-bye," I said.

I sat stunned for a few minutes. My eyes scanned the room and all I saw were a bunch of lucky bastards who did not just receive a cancer diagnosis. When my eyes eventually found the bar, I was snapped back to reality and realized my buddy was motioning me back over there. Yep, I think this called for a stiff drink or two.

Merkel Cell Diagnosis

While many experienced dermatologists can differentiate between basal cell and squamous cell carcinomas with a visual inspection, other lesions are more abnormal in appearance and most often require biopsy and microscopic study to confirm or rule out cancer.

A biopsy includes extraction of a small skin sample, typically by punch (a small core is taken) or shave (part of the top of the lesion is removed with a scalpel). This sample will be placed in a solution like formaldehyde, or in a sterile container. A pathologist will then study the immunohistochemistry stains under a microscope to determine the sample's characteristics.

The microscopic study will determine diagnosis. In the case of Merkel Cell Carcinoma, the sample will be positive for low molecular weight cytokeratins, or keratin proteins that are an important component in helping cells resist mechanical stress. Other indicators are necessary to confirm MCC diagnosis including the absence or presence of several other nuclear markers.

It is difficult to distinguish MCC from other small cell carcinomas. As such, electron microscopy and immunocytochemical studies are often required to correctly diagnose this type of cancerous tumor.

Pathologists will also perform a test to determine whether the sample includes the presence of the polyomavirus as it is present in 80% of MCC cases.

Chapter 3

Facing the Unknown

I barely slept the night I learned of my Merkel Cell Carcinoma diagnosis. A frantic Google search did not help. After reading various online articles in medical journals for about three hours followed by a few more stiff drinks, I couldn't believe this was my truth.

How would I explain this to my son? Do I even tell my son?

The next morning, I drove Dylan to school. I was still in shock and kept silent. Dylan was none the wiser and fiddled with the Bluetooth on his phone to get it to sync up with my car stereo. He loves music and his mother and I have always encouraged his interest in it. It's therapeutic and helps him focus and stay calm.

Dylan gave me a quick kiss on the cheek and a fast "Bye," as he ran from the car and into school.

I began to cry as my foot released the brake. But then the music abruptly stopped. Dylan was too far from the car now and his phone was out of range. He was gone. His music was gone. Would I be gone soon, too?

I turned the car onto the street heading west and stepped on the accelerator.

"Damn red light!" I yelled, wanting to drive as fast and far as possible. It was at that moment, sitting at a red light, that something funny happened.

There it was, a large dark shadow slowly moving through the intersection. Dozens of drivers were carelessly speeding through life and barely missed running it over.

Do I save the turtle? There was a line of cars behind me and this would certainly cause a delay.

The turtle was big, at least 50 pounds. A huge adult for sure. My life was uncertain that morning, but this turtle's life didn't have to be.

I jumped out of my car and quickly put my hands up to the drivers nearby. The light turned green but all lanes of traffic stopped. I could feel dozens of eyes fixed on my movements. I felt a little like Moses.

I approached the turtle and it immediately did what all turtles do when approached by humans, it stopped and recoiled into its shell. There was little time for introductions, people needed to get to work and I had to race the clock.

I hoisted the large reptile to my hips and moved briskly toward a guardrail. The turtle did what most turtles do when handled, it urinated and defecated on me. All over my nice suit pants and then it flowed down onto my best pair of shoes. A nice way to pay me back for saving its life.

I straddled the guardrail and nearly fell over it as the turtle's weight and my hold on it was beginning to shift. I was able to gently place the turtle at the water's edge of a retention canal that lined the road. It was safe. I had saved the turtle!

As I hopped over the guardrail with a feeling of accomplishment, I turned to look back at the turtle. He was crawling back out of the water and heading toward the rail. What a dummy, I thought! To have been saved and then choose to retrace the steps that put it in danger, what a dumb animal.

As I gave the universal "thumbs up" sign to drivers as a show of success, I noticed many of them taping my heroics with their cell phones.

Covered in turtle fear, I knew I'd have to move my morning appointments so I could go home and clean up. After a few quick calls to my clients, in which I regaled them with the story of the turtle rescue, I was heading back home with the windows open.

The song "Fantasy" by the band Earth Wind and Fire played on the car radio. It's one of my favorites and I turned the volume up as I sped past traffic on the highway.

It's your day, shining day, all your dreams come true
As you glide, in your stride with the wind, as you fly away
Give a smile, from your lips, and say
I am free, yes I'm free, now I'm on my way

A video of the rescue went viral on social media and to my surprise, was also featured on the local TV news that same evening.

Merkel Cell Carcinoma Treatment – Step 1: Surgery

Merkel Cell Carcinoma is an aggressive malignant neoplasm. A neoplasm is abnormal or excessive growth of a tissue.

Most scientific research concerning the initial treatment of MCC includes wide local excision of the primary lesion. In certain cases, especially those where the lesion is near a lymph node region, the surgeon may also perform a regional lymph node resection (removal).

For patients with stage I Merkel Cell Carcinoma, the tumor size is a predictor of survival. Recurrence of the disease occurs in 55% of these patients after surgical removal of the tumor, and the most common site of first recurrence is within a nearby lymph node.

The width of surgical margin around the primary site does not have a major impact on recurrence or survival rates.

In stage I and II Merkel Cell patients, lymph node removal is not typically performed.

In stage III patients, Merkel Cell has been detected in a regional lymph node and thus removal is warranted. This is called a lymphadenectomy.

After surgical removal of the tumor followed by radiotherapy, stage IV MCC patients remain at greatest risk of future nonlocalized metastases (the cancer indiscriminately spreads to other parts of the body).

Chapter 4

Saying Goodbye to Vanity

More money = more clients = more money = more work!

Once I found my passion lay in the financial planning field, I began collecting certifications like a Series 7 and insurance licenses and went to work for IDS (now Ameriprise). They trained me but I was captive to only sell their products and didn't like those restraints so I left and worked at an independent practice in Fort Myers where I could offer my clients more competitive solutions.

Working as a financial planner is hard work. It was the late 1990s and I was working days, nights and weekends so I decided to specialize. I spent three years studying to become a Chartered Financial Consultant® (ChFC®).

The next 10 years of my life were spent building my business in nearby Naples, Florida – one of the wealthiest communities in America.

It's hard to imagine but in 2001 the federal government would tax a person's estate that exceeded $600,000 at the time of death. I found a niche selling life insurance to cover the estate tax bill for clients. Even as the benchmark increased over the years, the concept was sound and my client roster grew.

During weekends I'd always be on the boat. Over time, I finally learned to barefoot water-ski on the Caloosahatchee River and was spending all my free time boating with friends.

One day I saw a guy skiing on his toes and approached him. His name was Randy Filter, and he was a national water ski champion. We became good friends and he taught me how to water-ski on my toes.

I was making great money but something was missing. I had been dating a nice lady and decided it was time to settle down and start a family.

I had been married briefly before; but like many first marriages, we were too young and too foolish.

I met Cori in the early 1990s at a friend's wedding. I was the best man and she was the maid of honor and our love was extraordinary. After dating for some time, she moved down from Sarasota and we were married for 22 years. We built a home together and our son Dylan was born in 2001.

Unfortunately, the odds are against married couples with autistic children. Nearly 85% of these marriages end in divorce, and ours was one of them. It was painful at first; but taking care of Dylan in two households is a better situation for everyone.

A Stitch in Time

I arrived early for my appointment with the surgeon. The doors were still locked so I sat in my car and listened to talk radio. It was time to turn lemons into lemonade. I was optimistic.

I checked in with the receptionist and took a seat near a tall fake ficus tree in the corner. Like most doctor's offices, there was a littering of magazines on various tables. My choices were *Men's Health*, *Better Homes & Gardens*, *Golf Digest*, *Florida Sportsman*, and a few local luxury lifestyles magazines. I grabbed a six-month-old issue of *Florida Sportsman* and began to page through it randomly. It's impossible to commit to a full article when you're waiting to meet a surgeon who is going to talk to you about removing a tumor, so I glanced at the pictures and advertisements.

Every page in the magazine reflected a lifestyle that was mine. The lifestyle I worked so hard to keep alive. Boating, fishing, and nature. I wanted to go back there again. Back to when I didn't give a care in the world about the consequences of not wearing a wide-brimmed hat. Back to a time when beer cans had pull tabs and bare feet replaced water skis.

The door swung open and a nurse assistant called my name. Reality check. I wasn't on my boat. I probably wouldn't be there anytime soon, but despite the seriousness of a surgical consultation ahead of me, I knew in my heart I would be there again someday with a full glass of lemonade.

I was led to a small patient room and left alone. After a few minutes, a surgeon entered. We spoke about nonconsequential topics like the weather for just a moment and then he performed a brief examination of the lesion. After removing the bright blue examination gloves and tossing them into a wastebasket, the surgeon turned to me and without fanfare told me surgery needed to happen as soon as possible.

Not soon after, on a foggy Friday morning, my friend George dropped me off at a surgery center near an upscale mall in southern Lee County where the surgeon removed the tumor and four lymph nodes.

The surgery took about two and a half hours. When I woke, the whole left side of my face hurt like hell. The surgery involved peeling back a large section of the skin from my hairline above my ear to my nose and down my neck. The tumor was the size of a small pearl.

A gel filler was used to rebuild a crater left on my temple from the surgery. It is amazing how well the gel can maintain facial form. The gel eventually disintegrates as the tissue regenerates.

I barely remember my friend Steve arriving to pick me up and drive me home.

My entire head was wrapped in white bandages and throbbed. I took one pain pill and went to bed. George visited me a few times over the weekend to make sure I was doing ok.

I met George and his wife while I was married and we became close friends. I'm glad he's still a good friend and didn't lose him in the divorce.

On Monday morning I returned to the surgeon's office where a nurse changed the bandage. I was shocked at the highway of stitches running across the side of my face and down my neck. There were 130 stitches in total!

The sun on my skin felt warm as I moved across the parking lot to my car. I was very aware of the physical feeling – but inside, it felt both peaceful and dreadful.

Would I ever enjoy the great outdoors the way I once did? And even if I lather my entire body with sunscreen, what are the chances the cancer will return? I'd read so much about MCC outcomes that I knew my future without cancer was not guaranteed.

Like many cancer survivors, a small fear of tomorrow lingers. Some days I'm Superman. Some days I'm Eeyore.

I decided to leave the bandages off so air could help the wound heal faster. Every night I placed Vitamin E oil on the stitches, and today you can barely see a scar.

To minimize his fear and avoid any painful discussions about my death, I told Dylan I had a cyst removed.

The surgeon had informed me that the biopsy results from the four lymph nodes he removed were positive for MCC so radiation would be an appropriate final step in my journey.

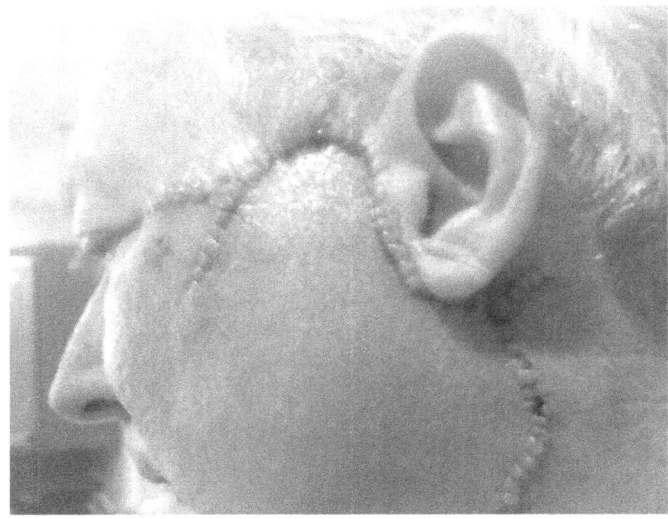

The trial of stitches on Pete's face after surgery to remove the Merkel Cell tumor on his temple.

At my follow-up appointment with the surgeon a few weeks later to remove all 130 stitches he asked me if I had made arrangements for radiation therapy.

I hadn't called the radiation oncologist at that point because I was scheduled for a full body scan at a local diagnostic imaging facility in a few days to see if there was cancer in other areas of my body.

The Cost of Cancer

When I got the MCC diagnosis in April, I had no health insurance. I had let my Blue Cross/Blue Shield policy lapse because the premiums were insanely high and I was healthy. This is behavior opposite to what I advise clients when discussing life insurance, but I thought I was the exception and not the rule.

God works miracles every day. One morning shortly after my diagnosis he provided me with a solution to the medical debt I was about to face. I was reading the newspaper and saw a story about a local kid who survived cancer. He had a tumor removed near his mouth and the doctor providing the care performed the surgery for free through a local Salvation Army program called WeCare.

I immediately picked up the phone and made the call to the Salvation Army office but got no answer. I called for days and finally decided to drive to downtown Fort Myers and sit in their office until someone would talk to me.

It worked and I spoke to a nice woman who listened to my story. I told her I had no health insurance and was just diagnosed with Merkel Cell Carcinoma. Not surprisingly, she had never heard of it so I educated her.

After about an hour of talking she leaned in close and said, "We'll cover the cost of it all."

WeCare is a program that coordinates specialty medical care for patients in need. I think it saved me $100,000 between the surgery, radiation therapy, and full body scans.

Because I had Stage III MCC that involved the lymph nodes, my prognosis was dire. In fact, my doctor deemed it terminal, and this allowed me to request an accelerated death benefit and pull out some money from a term life insurance policy to help cover living costs during my treatment and recovery.

Today, I have health insurance but I can't express the amount of comfort this program provided to me at a time when fear, stress, and pain were my bedfellows.

Merkel Cell Carcinoma Treatment – Step 2: Radiation

MCC is a radiosensitive cancer. Thus, in many cases of MCC, radiation therapy (radiotherapy) is used to destroy cancerous cells that remain after surgery has removed all clinically detectable tumors. Radiation therapy uses x-rays or similar forms of radiation to directly destroy cancer cells. It can also be used as a primary therapy in people for whom surgical removal of cancer is not possible. It is typically always prescribed when the cancer has spread to nearby lymph nodes (lymphovascular invasion).

Research has shown that radiotherapy improves local and regional recurrence rates for MCC. However, because MCC has a low incidence, very few, if any, controlled clinical trials are being done to study the outcomes of radiation therapy for MCC.

A review of 18 independent studies found that radiotherapy, when performed within weeks after excision of primary tumors or after surgical dissection for node-positive regional disease, reduces presence of the disease in the surgical bed. In these cases, radiotherapy after surgery was used to treat the potential residual disease and prevent disease progression.

Unfortunately, not enough data is available on surgery alone versus surgery and radiotherapy to accurately compare recurrence rates.

One study did investigate the association between the use of radiotherapy following surgical removal and overall survival in patients with MCC from 1973 to 2002. In 1,665 cases of MCC, 40% of the surgical patients were noted as having received adjuvant radiotherapy. The authors report that the median survival for patients receiving adjuvant radiotherapy was 63 months compared with 45 months for those treated with surgery alone.

Chapter 5:

There is No Escape Without Hope

Over the years I've had the good fortune to meet many wonderful people. Some of my closest friends are also clients. That's the essence of the life insurance business.

It's not a career for someone who doesn't understand the value of life.

To help a family create a financial future where they can live without worry is a huge responsibility. You have to invest in their lives, and not just a few hours but years! And you must be authentic in how you respond to their goals.

I've spent many happy holidays and weekends on and off the water with clients. A few of us will often charter a private jet to a football game. It's usually to a Vikings game.

In my career in the life insurance business, I've had 10 clients die from melanoma.

One of my dearest clients, who was also from Minnesota, was diagnosed with melanoma that metastasized and attacked his liver. I had sold him $6 million in life insurance to pay out to the family.

One day, he called me to discuss his premium payments on a $2 million policy I had sold him.

"Don't pay it," I said.

"Why not?" he asked.

"There's almost $300,000 in cash in there but the premium is $77,000," I answered. "If you die in the next few weeks, the insurance company will keep the $77,000 so keep your checkbook in your back pocket."

Instead I told him to make a three percent renewal on the policy. It lost me a commission, but it was the right thing to do.

I visited him several times in the hospital before he died.

I preach to people to buy life insurance when they are healthy for exactly this reason!

Cancer costs a ton of money; even if you have good health insurance or a social program that will help. I didn't have health insurance coverage at the time of my diagnosis but was fortunate to find a local non-profit that helped with the costs.

A Burning Gun at My Head

I met with a radiation oncologist in Fort Myers in mid-July to discuss his radiation treatment recommendations. He recommended a series of 30 treatments, starting immediately.

The first step in the radiation process is to create a mesh mold that goes over the head to keep it in place during the treatments. This involves laying a layer of warm flexible plastic mesh over the face. Straws are placed in the mouth and nose to ease breathing. As it cools, the mesh naturally forms to the face with a little extra work by a technician's hands.

I keep the mask in a closet now and it brings me great anxiety every time I bring it out to show a friend.

Late in the day on July 10th, I arrived at my first radiation therapy treatment. I didn't know what to expect or how long it would last, but I knew I'd be wearing that mask and I was already feeling scared. I was given a sedative but it made me groggy afterward so I refused them at future treatments.

The medical assistant helped me onto the treatment table and while affixing the mask must have sensed my apprehension because she calmly said, "It's ok, Pete. This is not going to be painful, you'll just feel a little heat on the side of your face."

I'm always surprised when people you don't know well tell you how to feel about something they've never experienced. How could she know how it would feel for me? She was in her 20s and it was highly unlikely that she ever had radiation.

One line in the lyrics of another Tom Petty song, "You don't know how it feels to be me," defines this experience perfectly. I felt alone when I first heard my diagnosis. But just like those friends I naturally accumulated through water-skiing, I began making new connections with a circle of people that had a very different common trait – they all experienced cancer.

In a short amount of time, and through compassionate humility, I had an army of new friends that understood how it feels. Their bravery and empathetic support helped me endure the toughest days in my cancer journey.

My first radiation treatment was actually uneventful and painless. I remember thinking, "This is nothing compared to the surgery." The treatments were scheduled daily and I'd go there after work. Each treatment took about seven or eight minutes total. The only bad thing about the radiation table is the annoying buzz of the machine and being strapped down with a mold over your face.

Each day I would arrive and sit in a waiting room filled with old men. After a few days I soon came to realize through idle conversations that most of them were getting radiation to treat advanced prostate cancer. It's the second most common cancer for men, after skin cancer. One in six men will have prostate cancer during his life.

But no one else there had MCC and most of the men I spoke with had never heard of it. Radiation therapy is often used as the primary treatment for prostate cancer.

Knowing what I already knew about the experience, I wondered what kind of mold they had to wear during treatment and how there was probably a cabinet filled with different sized molds for these other patients. The thought made me chuckle. Prostate molds?

At about the 15th radiation treatment I began to notice my mouth was very dry and there was a prominent permanent red mark on my temple and cheek.

I was originally scheduled to undergo a total of 30 radiation treatments but the doctor knocked it back to 25 soon after I began because initial results from early treatments were good.

After the 22nd treatment, I insisted on a break because the red spot had turned into a third-degree burn. I don't remember the doctor or medical assistant telling me *this* would happen. The burn was dark red with yellow edges and open sores that oozed. I was prescribed a special burn ointment.

The pain from the burn was incredible. I couldn't move my head to the right or tilt it backward. If I did, the skin would stretch and the blisters would reopen. Sleeping was impossible as my face and neck throbbed constantly.

I applied the ointment to my face for two weeks until the burn improved and pain subsided before reinitiating radiation treatments.

Afterburn Reactions

The women at the office were horrified when they saw the burns on my face from radiation. One of them even left the reception area in a hurry because of nausea from the sight.

I encountered many strangers' eyes peering in my direction when I was out in public after radiation. At the grocery store, the cashier had a look of disgust on her face that she couldn't hide. Even people in traffic would do a double take.

Through the years I've developed an ability to read people's body language. In all my sales interactions, this talent has been very useful. It's helped me detect reluctance from a client and then change my reaction or approach to help them become more at ease.

Typically, if I get the "crossed arms" signal from the wife of a client, then I immediately know that she's not ready to say "yes" because she doesn't understand how the recommended solution will help her.

I'm not upset by these reactions. I've been working in the financial services industry for more than 30 years now and it can be a complex process. Fortunately, all those years have provided me with great experience and that's how I can quickly determine what example to give, or story to tell, or question to ask.

Many salespeople don't put weight on the importance of patience and listening but I've found them to be the best sales tools in my toolbox.

I didn't have a whole lot of patience for cancer, though. Radiation had literally burned a hole in my face.

After two weeks off from the treatments, I set an appointment for August 13th and completed five more sessions. My goal was to be finished with cancer treatment before my birthday at the end of August.

That last week of radiation treatments was hell and I had three more to go but cancelled the appointments. The receptionist at the radiation therapy center called me several times to reschedule my final three treatments but the thought and pain was too severe for me to endure. I could barely move my head because the skin would stretch and reopen the burn sores. Despite the radiation oncologist's recommendation, I never returned for the final three radiation therapy treatments.

The radiation also caused problems with my left ear. After I ended the treatments, I sought out an ear, nose, and throat specialist. I met with an otolaryngologist but there was too much damage to my ear to place a tube in it. Instead, he evacuated a bunch of fluid from my ear and tested my hearing.

The pain in my ear returned after a week so I went to a nearby walk-in clinic and a physician assistant sucked out more fluid and what appeared to be hard black nuggets from my left ear.

Lethargy set in during the second week of radiation but I powered through it because I had clients to see and a kid to raise. My mouth was constantly dry so I drank gallons of water each day.

My appetite suffered, too. In the three months following radiation, I lost nearly 15 pounds. Nausea was also a side effect and vomiting became part of my daily routine.

My stomach hurt more after the sessions, too, so I went to a gastroenterologist and insisted on a colonoscopy. They found no polyps but identified several ulcers in my stomach. The doctor biopsied them but there was no cancer. He prescribed me Nexium and told me to severely limit my alcohol intake.

I ended up in the emergency room six times after radiation therapy ended to receive an IV of fluids due to dehydration. I couldn't take the nausea medication prescribed by my surgeon after radiation because I couldn't keep food down.

In November, I had another body scan done and it was clean again. Now that I was free from cancer, my last task was to improve my diet and vitamin intake. In addition to multivitamins I added milk thistle daily because radiation can cause damage to the liver. Heart disease runs in my family, so I take blood pressure medicine and statins daily. I also drink meal supplement shakes twice a day to give me some added protein and round out my diet.

When you boat a lot like I did you tend to navigate toward restaurants or bars that are on the water and that's where many of my regular meals were consumed. Not the healthiest foods admittedly. I'm cooking fresh meals at home now and feeling much better because of it.

Change is not always a negative. And sometimes it's a gift.

In my case, cancer helped me improve my overall health.

Merkel Cell Carcinoma Treatment – Step 3: Chemotherapy and Immunotherapies

According to the Skin Cancer Foundation, standard chemotherapy has never been tremendously beneficial for MCC patients.

It is often recommended only for patients whose cancer does not respond to immunotherapy (see below) or has spread to organs like the lungs or liver. A variety of chemotherapies have been used for advanced MCC with varied success. Unfortunately, no controlled clinical studies have shown that any of them extend survival, though they can often lead to short remissions.

An analysis of literature published over 15 years on the outcomes of 107 patients wherein chemotherapy was used to treat advanced MCC showed rare chemocurability in patients with metastasis or locally advanced tumors. The studies also reported a high incidence of toxic death due to chemotherapy.

However, for stage IV MCC patients, intravenous immunotherapy is showing great results. This type of treatment aims to enhance the body's innate ability to fight cancer using its own immune system.

As reported by the Skin Cancer Foundation, the U.S. Food and Drug Administration (FDA) approved the checkpoint blockade therapy drug avelumab (brand name Bavencio), for the treatment of adults and pediatric patients 12 years and older with MCC. The FDA based its approval on data from a clinical trial in which 33% of the patients experienced complete or partial shrinkage of their tumors.

Checkpoint blockade immunotherapies block certain molecules that inhibit or "check" T cell production to prevent excessive and potentially dangerous inflammatory and autoimmune reactions under normal conditions. By blocking these inhibiting molecules, the drugs release waves of T cells to attack the MCC cells.

Avelumab blocks programmed death-ligand 1 (PD-L1), a molecule that binds to another molecule called PD-1 (programmed death-1) on tumor cells, forming the complex that inhibits T cell activation. By blocking PD-L1, avelumab prevents it from binding with PD-1, thereby releasing T cells to fight MCC. In the avelumab trial, the responses lasted more than six months in 86% of responding patients and more than 12 months in 45% of responding patients.

Chapter 6:

Letting God Deliver Inner Strength

While the full body scans help identify whether new cancers are present, the process is not without discomfort as it involves an injection of dye (contrast) into the veins.

I must have been appeared visibly nervous when I arrived for my scan because the technologist, Addy, a nice, young woman told me a story that made me realize I was not alone. She had recently recovered from breast cancer and had a double mastectomy. During her treatment, she and her husband divorced and he left her with custody of their two young boys.

A few weeks later, I flew to Minneapolis to see a Minnesota Vikings game with Dylan and two close buddies. I had purchased four premium tickets from an online ticket vendor – but when we reached the entry gate – I was told the tickets were counterfeit.

It seemed our trip was a bust until I received a call from my surgeon while waiting in the airport security line.

"Hey Doc. I'm at the airport in Minnesota about to come home," I said and proceeded to tell him the unfortunate tale of our trip.

"Pete. Pete!" he interrupted finally. "The cancer didn't spread. The scan was clean, Pete. We got it all!"

The next day, I picked up a dozen roses and delivered them to Addy.

Finding Faith with God

Up until my MCC journey, I had very few health problems. Even hip surgery to repair an injury I suffered from a lifetime of water-skiing didn't create much fear because it didn't threaten my mortality like cancer.

A broken bone can be fixed, but cancer is a living organism. It wants to survive. I knew I had to prepare my mind and body for a future where cancer might return.

Shortly after my diagnosis I began attending church. Over the years, God had come in and out of my life, much like boats or cars. But with a cancer diagnosis, I knew I'd need more than just surgery. I knew it was bigger than me. I needed to build my heart up with God again and recover what faith I had lost over time.

Memories of my mother praying in desperate solitude was not the kind of religious experience that felt right for me so I opted to quietly visit Summit Church in Estero, Florida, and sit in the back with Dylan to observe.

It was not the kind of church experience I remembered as a child; one that involved prayerful incantations and sitting very still. The sermon at Summit was positive and uplifting and I was enveloped in the words of the songs and readings. I was hearing the gospel as an adult for the first time and it gave me a feeling of peace in my heart.

Faith is trust in God's future. No matter how much money I acquired, it could not guarantee a better tomorrow without God. I know this deep in my heart now.

I also know that God answers my prayers. It may not be the answer I had pictured but it's what God chooses. The Merkel Cell journey forced me to put aside my pride. I had to walk – my face disfigured – in public and receive judgment. I was forced to recognize that *"For our light and momentary troubles are achieving for us an eternal glory that far outweighs them all."* (2 Corinthians 4:17).

Shortly after my mother joined my father and brother, Tommy, in heaven, Cori found some of her old journals and gave them to me.

My mother was a voracious writer and documented everything in her journals, from her frequent trips to Minnesota to see my brother, Steve, and his family to the birth of her grandchildren and installation of new appliances in her home. But on every page (and in nearly every entry) she gives praise to God and Jesus.

"I pray I will do what's right in God's eyes," was her entry on Tuesday, December 15, 2009.

Her spirit and testament made me realize that I had to stop demanding or searching for ambition and become patient and appreciative of God's gifts. My beautiful boy, the smell of fresh coffee, the sounds of a choir, my place in His kingdom.

Reading my mother's journals has helped me become a humbler man and patient father. Her entries reciting Scripture touch me the most.

She wrote on Sunday, December 3, 2006: "Apostle Paul: 'I can do all things through Christ who strengthens me.'"

There is one entry in her journal that illustrates the kind of person she was and the kind of person we should all aspire to be.

On Saturday, October 6, 2001, my mother wrote: "In Old Testament, Book of Ecclesiastes, much wisdom given to us. We are all God's children, be content to help others, all are born, all die, seek truth, wisdom of God, be learned all our lives, we have happy times, and sad times, treasure our families, everyone and everything that is good."

Dylan loves to go to church, too. He especially likes to greet people as they exit the service. The benefits of renewing my faith have been extended to my child and this is doubly rewarding.

I can tell that Dylan feels encouraged by scripture and I know it will help him accept the challenges he may face when I am no longer by his side.

With scripture fresh in my heart and my mother's words in my ear, I find myself more giving of my time and money. One day in late April and shortly after my diagnosis, I approached a young man sitting outside a McDonald's in Fort Myers. He was homeless and seeking shelter. I asked him if he would accept my help and he agreed so we got in my car and I took him home.

His name was Gary and after a hot shower I gave him some fresh clothes and fed him at my club. He stayed in my guest room for a few nights and we watched the NBA playoffs together until my pastor could arrange shelter and job placement through a church ministry.

The recipe for my disaster was sun and fun. For others it's addiction and homelessness. But we are all God's children.

It's been almost a year since I received my MCC diagnosis but it seems like a lifetime ago.

Most of my physical fitness over the years involved activities on the water or outside during the heat of the day.

Today I'm avoiding the sun as much as possible. I used to golf weekly and water-ski every weekend. But now I stay fit using equipment inside a gym and watch my diet closely.

Most of my faith was buried in childhood but because of God's will, it's now alive in my heart again.

Beautiful Boy

I'm reading a terrific book right now called *Autism and the God Connection*, by William Stillman. I've read many, many books on autism and met many parents with autistic children over the last 16 years since we learned about Dylan's condition.

Stillman explains that autism "primarily affects one's ability to communicate in ways that are effective, reliable, and universally understandable."

We first recognized behavior that concerned us when Dylan was 18 months old. He would scoot across the floor on his back and shake his limbs erratically. It looked like he didn't have the motor control to stop it.

Over the next few years, we took him to a myriad of specialists including Pediatric Behavioral Specialists and Neurologists all across the country. We spent hundreds of thousands of dollars on therapies, consultations, observations and all manner of medical tests to help us understand the depth of his condition.

In the end, Dylan was diagnosed with autism and Asperger syndrome, which often manifests in obsessive behavior. It can be very difficult to redirect his attention but my sweet, beautiful boy is a gift and has given me a precious gift, too: He has helped me become a better person and advisor to clients because he taught me the power of patience.

I've also learned that autism is not a mental illness. Like most people, certain mental illness symptoms like anxiety and depression can surface temporarily from time to time. Dylan is sensitive and is not at the same level of social development as his peers. When he is with friends of the same age, he often struggles to manage his emotional reactions.

Dylan's therapy is not covered by insurance, but we will continue to utilize the services of autism therapists because we don't have all the answers and his needs are changing each year.

Unfortunately, his reading and writing skills are at a second-grade level, but his humor is very mature and he can get a group of grown men laughing in minutes. By law, he's able to stay in high school until he is 21 years old. He calls me every morning when he arrives at school and when the school day ends. He's my little buddy and likes to keep tabs on me and let me know how his day went.

Since the divorce, Dylan's behavior toward other women in my life has made dating a challenge for me.

When we are together, he demands my full attention and will often get verbally aggressive.

I have found that he enjoys simple tasks and often bring him to assist me at seminars. He likes to hand out or collect paperwork and shakes hands with everyone as they leave.

Since reconnecting with God and attending church, I have seen a profound change in Dylan's behavior that includes more moments of spiritual insight and compassion. He enjoys Bible stories and has memorized many. From time to time, he will describe a situation to me that happened in his day, and then, with pride, describe how it is similar to a story from the Bible.

Stillman explains that children with autism must be presumed to have intellect. I see this more and more in Dylan as he becomes a man and since returning to church services. Despite obstacles he may face with the disorder, Dylan's heart is pure and this fuels his capacity to grow his spiritual intellect. He may never write a graduate thesis, but he will also never suffer from a life void of God's gifts.

What's a Good Legacy?

Many financial advisors write a book to use as a marketing tool. They presume that a book will prove they are an authority on the subject and this will impress potential clients.

I've never written a book and never claimed to be an authority on any one subject. Until now.

I know what it's like to live through Merkel Cell Carcinoma. Moreover, now that my treatment is complete, I know I can help others avoid the same fate. I hope this book will inspire compassion and ignite support through the funding of more research so we can reduce the mortality rate of those who experience the disease in the future.

Unfortunately, talking about mortality is still taboo. But in my line of work, life and death is a necessary conversation topic. These two subjects are at the foundation of how I help people prepare financially for life's great moments and during times of crisis.

Life insurance is – by gross definition – money paid for death. I've faced death and I can honestly tell you that life insurance helped me survive. When I was unable to work, life insurance paid my bills. If I had died, life insurance would help my son's mother pay for his care. Life insurance can be a versatile tool, and the right policy can eliminate a lot of heartache and suffering.

During my career, I have learned two hard facts about people and their wealth: They want their principal investment intact and they want to earn income off it.

Actually, there are two more things they want: To avoid as much taxes as possible, and to leave money to children or charities.

One great tool to accomplish all of this is the Charitable Remainder Trust (CRT). However, it is best to seek the counsel of an estate planning attorney when setting up a CRT.

Here are the basics: Once a CRT is set up, you fund it by transferring assets into the trust. Then, these assets (like stocks or property) can be sold safely inside the trust, thus avoiding capital gains tax. The revenue from the sale is then invested in high-yielding investments and you enjoy a percentage payout (income).

The percentage payment must be at least 5% of the value of the assets within the trust. Be careful not to set your payout too high as a lower payout percentage provides for a larger tax deduction. But it depends on the investments. In several cases, I've been able to provide up to a 10% return.

The other advantage of this trust is that your principal is protected and will eventually benefit one or many named charities upon your death. You can even name a family foundation as one of the charities.

Once the last income beneficiary of the trust dies, the CRT's assets are distributed to the charities, and no estate taxes are due.

I have a client who held about $5 million in Coors (beer) stock. His initial investment was $450,000. When used to fund a CRT, we were able to sell the stock and avoid capital gains tax, a step-up in basis, fully fund a $1.6 million insurance policy, reinvest about $2.9 million in investments and annuities, and receive a $700,000 income tax deduction. Plus, he had a credit of $280,000 on his income tax for the next six years. In total, we saved him about $1.3 million doing it this way.

After advising another couple for years and helping them establish a sound estate plan, I told them, "It's time to spend all your money!" But the wife replied, "But we want to leave some to the kids." So instead of giving a lump $2 million in cash to the kids when they died, which would be taxable, I told them to purchase two life insurance policies. Their premium payments would be $20,000 a year for a $1 million policy with a long-term care rider and another $1 million second-to-die policy. We set them up in a CRT to eliminate some cost-basis issues and provide additional protections.

Life insurance is a great way to also remove the cost and threat of estate taxes from your estate upon your death. However, the estate tax exemption is $11.4 million per person so any wealth above this limit will be taxed at a rate of 40%.

There are two types of insurance: temporary and permanent. Term policies are temporary, have no cash value and are best for short-term needs. In some cases, they can be converted to permanent policies. Permanent insurance policies include whole life, universal life, indexed life, and variable life and have many benefits including flexible premiums and cash values.

Life insurance proceeds are free of income tax – but not federal estate taxes – unless the insured is not the owner. However, when a life insurance policy is placed in an Irrevocable Life Insurance Trust (ILIT), certain protections from estate taxes apply.

ILITs are extremely useful as they remove assets from an individual's estate while providing some degree of control.

Upon death, proceeds from the insurance policy inside the trust are used to pay for any estate taxes owed.

For example, I had a client whose husband died and left her with three small kids. She was the beneficiary on a $5 million life insurance policy. As a young, attractive newly-widowed woman, she became the object of very unscrupulous men and met a gigolo. Unfortunately, he went through her $5 million in three years. Had it been in an

ILIT it would have been protected from predators like this man.

I've set up two policies so my son will be cared for when I am gone. The first ILIT policy pays out $1.5 million in trust for Dylan's care into adulthood. Another $2 million policy lists my ex-wife as beneficiary so she can access any money she needs to care for him as well. I've also set up another $1 million policy on Cori for Dylan when she dies. The premiums are low because I bought them six years ago when I was healthy.

For years until recently, I gave educational seminars on the benefits of ILITs and estate planning at luxury hotels or fine restaurants often providing entertainment and serving meals. The rooms were packed and business thrived.

My marketing strategy included direct mail and full-page advertisements in the daily newspaper. This worked very well until the planner market tripled and financial seminars in my town became as frequent as sunsets.

When the estate tax rate was low, my seminars were packed. But any couple who has more than $20 million in assets isn't going to seminars today. They have teams of professionals that manage everything. So now my marketing strategy is to build relationships with other financial planners, estate planning attorneys, and CPAs, and educate them on the benefits of ILITs.

And because my services best serve families that have assets of $1 million and more, that's who gets most of my in-office counsel today.

But I believe, as the Bible teaches, that God shows no partiality so I will continue to host free public seminars. This way, anyone can attend and learn how to protect their financial future, regardless of the size of their bank account.

Hope Brings Promise to Tomorrow

I know my future includes more skin cancer but not necessarily MCC. I'll continue to see Beth at Riverchase Dermatology regularly over the next year and get body scans every six months until my last day on earth.

My internist was also a close ally during my journey through MCC and his guidance and care was instrumental after radiation.

Long-term effects of radiation included pain in my neck, which turned out to be a problem with my vertebrate. The radiation oncologist suggested physical therapy so I make regular visits to a physical therapist to address the pain.

Now that I'm not drinking alcohol regularly, my blood pressure is good. The ulcer problems are also reduced because of the reduced drinking. Booze has lots of sugar and cancer loves sugar so its removal from my diet is a good thing.

Sugar intake also caused health problems with my younger brother, who now lives with diabetes and takes insulin daily.

In December 2018, the FDA granted accelerated approval to a second immunotherapy, pembrolizumab (brand name Keytruda), for patients with recurrent locally advanced or metastatic MCC. Pembrolizumab was previously approved for treatment of advanced melanoma patients, whose lives it has sometimes extended by many years, sending the disease into long-term remission.

Pembrolizumab blocks the immune-inhibiting molecule PD-1, thereby releasing waves of T cells to attack the cancer cells. As 64% of the responding patients in this study had the Merkel cell polyomavirus, it suggests that antigens from the virus may have enhanced therapeutic response. Future studies will investigate whether pembrolizumab and other treatments can indeed target the polyomavirus.

Sharing the Hope

Like many people who are touched by a life-altering medical event, I feel a strong responsibility to advocate for those suffering from terminal skin cancer. This book and its proceeds will help fund ongoing and future research that develops new treatments, care, and a better understanding of MCC.

My journey has been unique and my story has already been featured by several local media. I'm currently negotiating an appearance on a national, highly rated medical advice television show and I've been asked to write a blog about my journey and the advocacy work I am doing on the Skin Cancer Foundation's website.

It's been a year since my diagnosis and I am a different man. I recently spoke to more than 500 kids at a local high school about the dangers of sun damage and how to avoid skin cancer later in life. Most of them are just like I was when I was young: innocent and invincible. But they have something I didn't have that may change the way they behave toward cancer: access to a wealth of information in their pocket.

While 100% of the high school students I spoke to had never heard of Merkel Cell Carcinoma when I took the stage, by the end of my presentation a majority of them had done a quick internet search on the topic. With the help of great organizations such as the Skin Cancer Foundation, I have no doubt that future generations will be better armed with good information that can save their lives.

I will continue to advocate the importance of regular check-ups with a dermatologist and how to take steps to reduce the possibility of a future with skin cancer. That said, I am available to speak to any group about my journey for free.

"He that findeth his life shall lose it: and he that loseth his life for My sake shall find it." (Matthew 10:39 King James Version)

If you would like to see more studies done on Merkel Cell Carcinoma, please consider making a donation to the Skin Cancer Foundation. I am also happy to talk to you about how you can maximize your charitable contributions by using life insurance and trusts.

Bibliography

In writing *There is Hope! Surviving Merkel Cell Carcinoma*, I supplemented the accounts of my own experiences with supporting data from the following published resources.

Chapter 1:
American Cancer Society. Cancer.org. What is Melanoma Skin Cancer?

Grabowski, Julia, et. al. "A Comparison of Merkel Cell Carcinoma and Melanoma: Results from the California Cancer Registry." *Clinical Medicine: Oncology.* 2008; 2: 327-333.

Hodgson, NC. "Merkel cell carcinoma: changing incidence trends." *Journal of Surgical Oncology.* 2005; Jan 1; 89(1):1-4.

Martinez VD, et al: "Arsenic exposure and the induction of human cancers." *Journal of Toxicology.* 2011; 431287.

Schmerling, Rafael A., et al. "Burden of Disease, Early Diagnosis, and Treatment of Merkel Cell Carcinoma in Latin America." *Journal of Global Oncology.* 2018

Toker C. Trabecular carcinoma of the skin. *Cancer.* 1978; 105:107-110.

Chapter 2:

Ratner, D. Nelson, et al. "TM Merkel cell carcinoma: continuing medical education." *Journal of the American Academy of Dermatology*. 1993; Volume 29:143-156.

Riverchase Dermatology, Riverchasedermatology.com

Seattle Cancer Care Alliance, University of Washington MCC Research, Merkelcell.org

Sur, Monalisa, et al. "TdT expression in Merkel cell carcinoma: potential diagnostic pitfall with blastic hematological malignancies and expanded immunohistochemical analysis." *Modern Pathology*. 2007; Volume 20, pages 1113-1120.

Chapter 3:

Allen, P.J., Zhang, Z.F., and Coit, D.G. "Surgical management of Merkel cell carcinoma." *Annals of Surgery*. Jan; 229(1): 97–105. (1999).

Banks, Patricia D., et al. "Recent Insights and Advances in the Management of Merkel Cell Carcinoma." *Journal of Oncology Practice*. 2016; Volume 12, No. 7, 637-646.

Gillenwater, Ann M. et al. "Merkel Cell Carcinoma of the Head and Neck Effect of Surgical Excision and Radiation on Recurrence and Survival." *Otolaryngology Head Neck Surgery*. 2001; 127(2):149-154.

Chapter 4:

Mojica, P., Smith, D., Ellenhorn JD. "Adjuvant radiation therapy is associated with improved survival in Merkel cell carcinoma of the skin." *Journal of Clinical Oncology*. 2007; 25(9):1043–1047.

Rush, Zoe, et al. "Radiation therapy in the management of Merkel cell carcinoma: current perspectives." *Expert Review Dermatology*. 2011; 6(4): 395–404.

Chapter 5:

Nghiem, Paul T., et al. "PD-1 Blockade with Pembrolizumab in Advanced Merkel-Cell Carcinoma." *The New England Journal of Medicine*. 2016; 374:2542-2552

Skin Cancer Foundation, skincancer.org/skin-cancer-information/merkel/treatment

Chapter 6:

www.merkelcell.org (a public resource from the Seattle Cancer Care Alliance)

Skin Cancer Foundation, skincancer.org

How to Contact Peter D. Jepson

Office: (239) 263-2204

Email: peterjepson@mindspring.com

Website: www.peterdjepson1.com

This book is available for purchase
through major online booksellers
including Amazon and at
www.peterdjepson1.com.

Complimentary copies are available
to clients of Riverchase Dermatology,
upon request.

www.ingramcontent.com/pod-product-compliance
Lightning Source LLC
Chambersburg PA
CBHW071120280526
45787CB00003B/1115